Understanding Medical Terminology

A Reference to Help You Learn and Memorize Medical Terminology

By S.W. Livingston

Text Copyright © 2019 S.W. Livingston

All Rights Reserved

No part of this book may be reproduced

in any way without the written

permission of the author.

Disclaimer:

The views expressed within this book are those of the author alone. The information contained within this book is based on the opinions, experiences, and observations of the author and is provided "AS-IS". No warranties of any kind are made. Neither the author nor publisher are engaged in rendering professional services of any kind. Neither the author nor publisher will assume liability or responsibility for any loss or damage related directly or indirectly to the information contained within this book.

The author has attempted to be as accurate as possible with the information contained within this book. Neither the author nor publisher will assume responsibility or liability for any errors, omissions, inconsistencies, or inaccuracies.

Table of Contents

Introduction 1
How to Improve Your Memory 3
Medical Terms and their Meanings 6
A 6
B 10
C 11
D 14
E 15
F 17
G 17
H 19
I 20
J 21
K 21
L 22
M 23
N 24
O 25
P 25
Q 27
R 27
S 28
T 30
U 32
V 32
W 33
X 33
Y 33
Z 33
Body Systems 34
Closing 36

Introduction

The medical language can seem a bit overwhelming at first, but it doesn't have to be scary. Although the risk of miscommunication between medical coders and doctors is present, this risk can be minimized when proper training is utilized.

Part of the training process includes an ability to understand and memorize medical terminology.

Medical terminology includes—but is not limited to—terms that describe a number (mono, uni, etc), where a condition or procedure takes place in the body (ecto, endo, etc), and conditions that may affect certain body parts (Eukaryote, Sleep apnea, etc).

Many of these terms will include a prefix, a root word, and a suffix. Although memorizing every single medical term may not be realistic, it is important to memorize as many as you can to help prevent as many errors and misunderstandings as possible.

One way of memorizing a large number of medical terms is by learning the most popular prefixes and suffixes for some of the most popular root words.

To illustrate, memorizing the meaning of the suffix, "ITIS" which means, "inflammation", can give you the ability to have at least a partial understanding of a large number of medical terms.

This is because whether someone uses the term, "Tendinitis" or "Bronchitis", you will already know that it has something to do with the inflammation of a particular body part. You will have provided yourself with a foundation to work with.

Whether you plan to work in the medical field or are simply interested in learning medical terminology, this book can help.

It will include an alphabetized list of medical terms, as well as information on how to effectively memorize as many of them as you can.

How to Improve Your Memory

Before getting to the medical terms and their meanings, it can be beneficial to understand how to maximize your ability to memorize them.

Looking up a word and its meaning can help you in the *short* term, but memorizing the word and its meaning can help you in the *long* term.

Creating Associations

One of the best ways to memorize a term is by associating it with something that stands out in your mind.

The association can simply be another word that helps you connect the pieces of the puzzle together, so to speak.

To illustrate, the word, "cranium," might remind a person of the word, "crane." Now that person must simply find a way to connect the word, "crane" with the word, "cranium."

Since the word, "cranium" means the skeleton of the head, which holds the brain, that person can creatively picture a crane loading a brain into a skeleton and holding it there. Another benefit of the word, "crane" in this example is that it rhymes with the word, "brain," which can make the example easier to memorize.

The fact that cranes do not load brains into skeletons is irrelevant. What matters is whether or not it helps the person memorize the meaning of the word.

In fact, the more unusual the example is, the more likely the person is to remember it.

If the initial example the person comes up with does not seem to help him or her remember the meaning of the term, another example can be sought.

Keep brainstorming until you find an example that works.

Repetition

After reliable associations are established, its best to repeat them to yourself to ensure that the terms and their meanings stay in your memory.

They can be repeated out loud or in your head, although out loud is typically best.

The repetitions don't even have to be complete sentences. Using the same example from earlier, you might say, "Cranium = crane. Crane rhymes with brain. Crane = place brain in skull."

If successful, you will remember that the cranium's function is to hold the brain.

To make sure that the information is staying in your memory, try testing yourself by gradually increasing the time periods between sessions while decreasing the practice sessions.

For example, practice the repetitions for fifteen minutes every hour. Then practice the repetitions for ten minutes every other hour. Next, practice the repetitions for just five minutes every twenty-four hours, and so forth.

* * *

By breaking the process down into a series of small steps, you can effectively memorize just about anything you choose to.

It's a matter of combining creativity and consistency.

Medical Terms and their Meanings

This is not intended to be an entirely inclusive list of medical terminology. The intention is to have a list of medical terms that are the most likely to be used in the medical field, while excluding some of the more obvious ones that many people already know the meaning of.

For example, since many people are already familiar with the term, "medicine" and it's meaning, a word such as that may be excluded from this list.

A

Abdomen: The portion of the body cavity that is located below the thorax.

Abdominal aorta: The portion of the aorta that passes through the diaphragm into the abdomen.

Abdominal quadrants: Four portions of the abdomen that are divided by imaginary horizontal and vertical lines.

Abdominal thrusts: Also known as the Heimlich Maneuver. A procedure that is applied to relieve choking. It involves a thrusting of the hands in an inward and upward motion toward the diaphragm.

Abdominal wall: The lining of the abdomen, consisting primarily of muscle but also some bone.

Abdominoplasty: Cosmetic surgery of the abdomen that involves the removal of excess skin and fat.

Abducens nerve: A cranial nerve that controls the movement of the lateral rectus muscle, which is responsible for the outward gaze of the eye.

Abduction: Movement of a limb away from the midline or axis of the body.

Aberration: A departing from a normal condition or behavior.

Ablation: Removal or destruction of tissue through surgery.

Abreaction: An emotional release after recalling a repressed experience.

Abscess: A collection of pus that is often accompanied by swelling and inflammation.

Accessory nerve: A cranial nerve that provides control for certain neck muscles.

Acetabulum: A part of the pelvis where the head of the thighbone is.

Achilles tendon: A tendon that attaches the muscles in the calf to the bone of the heel.

Acidosis: Abnormal condition that occurs when there is an excess of acid in the body.

Actinic keratosis: A pre-cancerous patch of thick, scaly, or crusty skin that forms after years of sun exposure.

Actinomycosis: A long-term bacterial disease that typically affects the face and neck.

Acupuncture: A type of therapy that is used for treating pain or disease. It involves the use of needles that are inserted along specific points.

Acute: Happening suddenly with severity and lasting a short time.

Adduction: Movement of a limb toward the midline of the body.

Aden(o): Gland.

Adentitis: Inflammation of a lymph node.

Adenoids: Enlarged lymphoid tissue at the back of the pharynx.

Adhesion: Strands of scar tissue that can form after surgery.

Adnexa: Appendage of an organ.

Adrenal: Pertaining to the adrenal glands, which are located at the top of the kidneys.

Aer-: Air.

Aerobics: Cardiovascular exercise.

Aftercare: Healthcare that is offered to a patient after discharge.

Ageusia: Inability to taste.

Agnosia: Inability to comprehend or recognize the significance of a variety of stimulation.

-agra: Pain that is severe.

Airway: The passage through the throat that carries air to the lungs.

Alexia: Inability to read.

-algia: Pain.

Algid: Cold.

Alkalosis: Excessive alkalinity of the blood and tissues.

Allograft: Transfer of a tissue or organ from individual to another of the same species with different genetics.

Alopecia: Disorder that causes hair loss.

Alveoli: Small air sacs at the end of bronchioles.

Ambulatory: Having the ability to walk; not bedridden.

Amino acid: Building blocks of proteins.

Analgesia: Absence of pain, even though the patient is conscious.

Andro-: Male.

Andropause: Male version of menopause.

Aneurysm: Dilation of a blood vessel, which could be a sign that the wall may rupture.

Angina Pectoris: Chest pain that is caused by a lack of oxygen to the heart muscle.

Anterior: Front.

Aorta: The largest artery in the body, which carries blood from the left ventricle of the heart to other parts of the body.

Aplasia: Incomplete or faulty development in an organ or tissue. The organ or tissue may be defective or missing entirely.

Apnea: Temporaryabsence of breathing.

Asphyxia: Lack of oxygen, which leads to loss of consciousness and death, such as by choking.

Atonic: Absence of normal muscle tone or strength.

Atria: Upper chambers of the heart.

Atrium of the heart: chamber of the heart that leads to the ventricle.

Atrophy: Reduction in size or wasting away of body tissue.

Autoimmune disorder: An attack on healthy cells by the immune system.

Autopsy: Postmortem exam of the body that is used for the purpose of determining the cause of death.

Avascular: Having little to no blood vessels.

B

Ballism: Abnormal movements.

Bar(o): Weight.

Bariatric: Relating to the treatment of obesity.

Basal Cell Carcinoma: A type of skin cancer that is typically is not fatal and rarely spreads to other body parts.

Benign: Non-cancerous.

Bio: Life.

Biofeedback: A technique that utilizes a monitor to read a patient's physiological information.

Biopsy: Removal of a piece of tissue from a body for the purpose of sending it to the lab for examination.

Blackhead: A small, dark spot on the skin due to a blocked pore.

Blood count: The determination of the number of red and white blood cells and platelets in a particular volume of blood.

Blood sugar: The concentration of glucose in the blood.

Body Mass Index: A formula that uses the height and weight of a person to determine that person's level of obesity.

Boil: An inflamed, tender portion of skin that contains pus.

Bone density: A measure of the amount of minerals that are found in a certain volume of bone.

Bone marrow: Soft vascular tissue that fills the cavities of bones. It contains fat and blood cells.

Bougie: A thin cylinder of material that a doctor inserts into or through body canals for examination purposes.

Brachial: Relating to the arm.

Brachial artery: Artery that lies between the shoulder and the elbow.

Brachytherapy: A type of radiation therapy in which radioactive material is placed near or directly into a tumor.

Bradycardia: Cardiac arrhythmia that is characterized by abnormally slow heart rate. For adults, this is typically below 50 bpm.

Bradykinesia: Abnormally slow body movement.

Bradypnea: Slow breathing.

Buccal: Relating to the mouth or inner cheek.

Bulla: An elevated lesion with a blister-like appearance, typically measuring more than 5mm in diameter.

C

Calcitonin: A hormone that helps regulate calcium levels and is secreted by the thyroid gland.

Caliper: A tool with two adjustable arms that measures diameter or thickness. For example, calipers can be used to measure body fat near the waistline.

Canal: A tubular passageway.

Capillaries: Small blood vessels that distribute oxygen and nutrients to cells.

Carbon dioxide: A colorless gas that passes through the lungs before being exhaled.

Carbon monoxide: A highly toxic colorless gas that has no scent or taste.

Carcin(o): Cancer.

Cardiovascular system: Refers to the heart and blood vessels.

Carotene: A red or yellow organic compound that is found in certain types of foods.

Carpal: Relating to the wrist.

Cartilage: Rubbery tissue that acts a cushion for the joints in the bones.

Casein: A type of protein found in milk.

Cat-scratch fever: A bacterial infection that results from a feline scratch.

Cataract: A loss of transparency of the eye lens caused by tissue breakdown and clumping of protein.

Caustic: Substance that destroys living tissue.

Celiac: Relating to the abdominal cavity.

Central nervous system: Consists of the brain, spinal cord, and meninges.

Cerebellum: Part of the brain that is located in the posterior base of the skull, and is used to coordinate voluntary muscle activity, balance and tone.

Cerebral contusion: A bruising of brain tissue.

Cerebrum: The largest, uppermost part of the brain that is responsible for initiating and controlling voluntary movements.

Chalazion: A small tumor of the eyelid caused by a blocked oil gland.

Chemotherapy: The use of chemicals to treat cancer.

Chorea: A disorder that is characterized by spasmodic movements.

Choroid: Thin, vascular layer that runs from the retina to the sclera.

Chronic: Prolonged.

Chronic fatigue syndrome: A disorder characterized by extreme tiredness that is not relieved with rest.

Chronic obstructive pulmonary disease: Respiratory disease that affects bronchial air movement.

Circadian: Occurring in approximately 24-hour periods.

Cirrhosis: A chronic liver disease characterized by scarring.

Clavicle: Collar bone.

Collagen: A group of fibrous proteins that is found in the skin, tendons, cartilage, bone, and connective tissue.

Colon: Main part of the large intestine.

Congenital heart defect: An abnormality of the heart that is present at birth.

Congestion: Occurrence of abnormal levels of fluids in an organ or vessel.

Congestive hear failure: An inability of the heart to pump enough blood.

Conjugate: Joined.

Constriction: Abnormal narrowing of an opening.

Convulsion: A type of seizure.

Cornea: The anterior part of the eye, which is the eye's main refractory structure.

Coronary artery: Supplies blood to the heart muscles from the aorta.

Cortex: Outer layer of a structure.

Costal: Relating to the ribs.

Cranium: Skeleton of the head that holds the brain.

Crohn's disease: Chronic inflammation of the gastrointestinal tract.

Cubital: Relating to the elbow or forearm.

___D___

Debribement: Removal of dead, damaged, or contaminated substances from a wound.

Defibrillation: The application of electric shock to a patient's chest to restore the normal cardiac rhythm.

Delirium: A state of confusion that can sometimes be accompanied by hallucinations.

Deltoid: Should muscle.

Dementia: Loss of remembering, reasoning, and thinking skills.

Dentin: Main material of the teeth.

Depersonalization: A feeling of disconnection from reality.

Dermatology: Medical specialty that focuses on the skin.

Desiccation: The removal of moisture from a substance.

Dialysis: The removal of excess fluid from the body when the kidneys are not functioning optimally.

Diaphragm: Sheet of muscle that separates the abdomen from the thoracic cavity.

Diastolic blood pressure: The second number in blood pressure readings.

Diplopia: Double vision.

Disorientation: A state of mental confusion.

Dissociation: A state in which the patient has a disconnection from his or her own thoughts, memory, and sense of identity.

Dopamine: A neurotransmitter in the brain.

Dyslexia: A condition that impacts the way the brain processes written and verbal language.

Dystrophy: A condition that results from poor nutrition.

E

Echocardiography: The examination of the heart through the use of ultrasound. It is a non-invasive procedure.

Ecto-: Outward.

Ectomorph: A very lean body type. An person with an ectomorph body type typically has a fast metabolism.

-ectasis: Stretching.

-ectomy: Excision.

Edema: Swelling as a result of excessive fluid in body tissue.

Electrocardiography: A procedure that records the electrical activity of the heart.

Electroencephalography: A procedure that measures the electrical activity of the brain.

-emia: Blood condition.

Emphysema: A chronic lung disease that can be caused by genetic defects or smoking.

Endo-: Inward.

Endocrine system: System of glands that release hormones into the circulatory system.

Endomorph: A soft and round body type. A person with an endomorph body type typically has a slower than average metabolism.

Endorphin: A naturally-occurring substance produced in the brain that react with opoid receptors.

Endoscope: A tool that is used for visual examination of the body's interior.

Epilepsy: Recurring seizures.

Erythema: Reddening of the skin caused by capillary congestion.

Excision: The removal of tissue by using a scalpel.

Exfoliation: The removal of a skin layer.

Exocrine glands: Glands that secrete to the body's cavities, surface, or organs.

F

Femoral: Relating to the thigh.

Femur: The largest bone of the skeleton, located between the knee and the hip.

Fibrillation: Rapid twitching of muscle fibers due to abnormal electrical impulses.

Fibroma: A benign tumor that consists of fibrous tissue.

Fibromyalgia: A chronic disorder characterized by musculoskeletal pain, fatigue, and issues with sleep, memory, and mood.

Fissure: A small tear.

Fistula: An abnormal passageway in the body.

Flexor: A muscle that causes a limb to bend.

Follicle: A small bodily cavity.

Forceps: An instrument that is used to firmly hold tissues.

Formication: A type of hallucination in which patients feel like there are bugs crawling on their skin.

Frontal bone: A bone that makes up the forehead and the upper edge and roof of the eye socket.

G

Galactose: A simple sugar found in the protein of milk.

Ganglion: A cluster of nerve cell bodies found in the peripheral nervous system.

Gangrene: Localized death of soft tissue caused by a loss of blood supply.

Gene: A sequence of nucleotides that is typically located on a chromosome. It is the basic physical unit of heredity.

Geni(o): Chin.

Genosome: Complete group of genes in the chromosomes of each cell.

Ger(o): Old age.

Geriatrics: Medical branch that specializes in the elderly.

Gestation: Time period from fertilization to the actual birth.

Gigantism: Abnormal growth of the body, often due to a dysfunctional pituitary gland.

Gingiva: Gums.

Glabella: The area that is directly above the nose and between the eyebrows.

Glandular: Relating to the glands.

Glaucoma: An eye disease that is often due to abnormally high pressure in the eye.

Gleason score: Grading system that classifies malignancy of prostate cancers.

-globin: Containment of protein.

Glucose: The main sugar that the body manufactures. It is located in the blood and is the primary source of energy.

Glyc(o): Glucose.

Glycemic index: Numerical system that is used to measure how carbohydrates affect blood glucose levels.

Glycine: A non-essential amino acid.

Goiter: A swelling in the front of the neck, caused by an enlargement of the thyroid gland.

Gout: Acute arthritis.

-gram: Recording.

Granulation tissue: Connective tissue and blood vessels that form on the surfaces of a wound during the healing process.

-graph: Recording instrument.

-graphy: Recording process.

Gynecomastia: A non-cancerous swelling of the chest tissues in males, caused by a hormonal imbalance.

H

Heart block: A blockage in the process of normal electrical impulses in the heart.

Heart murmurs: Sounds caused by vibrations of the blood flow through the heart.

Heart valves: Thin tissues that open and close to allow blood to flow through the heart.

Hematology: Medical branch that specializes in blood diseases.

Hemoglobin: Oxygen-carrying pigment in red blood cells.

Hernia: Protrusion of an organ caused by weakness of a muscle and strain.

Heterophoria: A condition in which one eye deviates from the other at the fixation point.

Histamine: A substance that regulates physiological function in the gut, acts as a neurotransmitter for the brain, spinal cord, and uterus, and is released in allergic inflammatory reactions.

Histogram: Bar chart.

Histology: Study of tissue structure with a microscope.

Holography: Method of recording three-dimensional images.

Homeostasis: Process of maintaining physiological balance.

Hospice: Facility that provides care for terminally-ill patients.

Humerus: Upper arm bone.

Huntington disease: A progressive disorder that is usually inherited and causes neurons to die.

Hyperopia: Farsightedness.

I

Ileum: The narrowest portion of the small intestine.

Ilium: The largest of three bones composing each half of the pelvic girdle.

Impetigo: A contagious skin disease that typically affects infants and children.

Impingement syndrome: An impingement of tendons in the shoulder.

Incision: A surgical cut.

Infarction: Death of tissue caused by a lack of oxygen.

Inflammation: Swelling, redness, pain, or a feeling of heat due to infection, irritation, or injury.

Influenza: Contagious viral infection of the respiratory system.

Infusion pumps: Device that transfers intravenous fluids.

Insomnia: Inability to get to sleep or stay asleep.

Insulin: A hormone that regulates glucose levels.

Intubation: Insertion of a tube.

Iodine: An element and essential nutrient in the diet.

Iris: Membrane behind the cornea that gives the eye its color.

Irrigation: The washing out of a wound.

-itis: Inflammation.

J

Jaundice: Yellow staining of the skin and whites of the eyes.

Joints: The points of connection located between the ends of the bones.

Jugular veins: Major veins that moves blood from the head to the heart.

K

Keloid: An overgrowth of scar tissue .

Keratin: A group of fibrous proteins that are the basis of the epidermis.

Ketosis: The state in which the body utilizes fats for energy instead of glucose.

L

Laceration: A deep tear of the skin.

Lactase: An enzyme that converts lactose into glucose and galactose.

Lactic acid: An organic liquid that is produced to muscle contraction, especially anaerobic respiration.

Lactose: The main sugar in milk.

Lapar/o: Abdominal wall.

Larynx: Voice box, which includes the vocal cords.

Later/o: Side.

Lateral: Away from the body's midline.

Lesion: Abnormal change or damage to tissues.

Lethargy: State of fatigue or lack of energy.

Leukemia: Blood cancer.

Leukocyte: White blood cell.

Ligament: A fibrous band of tissue that connects the extremities of bones to form a joint.

Limbic: Edge.

Lipids: Fats.

Lumbar: Relating to the lower back.

Lupus: A chronic autoimmune disease that can cause damage to any part of the body.

Lyme disease: Inflammatory disorder that is typically transmitted by ticks. The initial sign of the disease is a red rash at the bite site, followed by flu-like symptoms.

Lymph node: A part of the body's immune system.

Lysine: An essential amino acid.

M

Macro-: Large.

Macul/o: Spot.

Macular degeneration: Loss of vision in the center of the visual field.

Madarosis: Underdevelopment or loss of eyebrows or eyelashes.

Mal-: Bad.

Malaise: An overall feeling of illness.

Medial: Relating to the middle.

Medulla: Inner area of a body structure or organ.

-megaly: Enlargement.

Melatonin: A hormone that helps regulate sleep, reproduction, and mood.

Membrane: Thin layer of tissue that covers a surface.

Meninges: The three membranes that coat the brain and spinal cord.

Menopause: Time period in which menstruation stops permanently.

-Mer: Partial.

Mes-: Middle.

Mesomorphic: Muscular body type.

Mio-: Smaller.

Mitral valve: A valve located between the left ventricle and left atrium of the heart.

Morbid: Unhealthy or diseased.

Morph/o: Shape or form.

Mort/o: Death.

Myalgia: Muscle pain.

Myopia: Nearsightedness.

N

Narc/o: Stupor.

Narcolepsy: Chronic sleep disorder characterized by extreme daytime drowsiness and sudden onsets of sleep.

Nas(o): Nose.

Natal: Pertaining to birth.

Necr-: Death.

Neo-: New.

Nephr(o)-: Kidney.

Nerve: Bundle of fibers that use electrical and chemical signals to transmit information between the brain and other body parts.

Neur(o)-: Nerve.

Noct/i: Night.

O

Ocul/o: Eye.

Odont/o: Tooth.

Olfactory: Pertaining to the sense of smell.

Olig(o): Few, little.

Onco-: Tumor.

Onych/o: Nail.

Ophthalm(o): Eye.

Opt(o): Vision.

Optic nerve: Cranial nerve that transmits visual information from the retina to the brain.

Orth(o): Straight, correct.

-osis: Abnormality.

Oss(e): Bone.

Ot(o): Ear.

-ous: Relating to.

P

Pacemaker: System that transmits electrical impulses to the heart for the purposes of setting a heart rhythm.

Palate: Roof of the mouth.

Pancreas: A gland located behind the stomach that secretes digestive enzymes, insulin, and glucagon.

Para-: Beside.

Path(o): Disease.

Pelvis: Structure in the skeleton that is located near the pelvic girdle and the connecting bones of the spine.

-penia: Lack or deficiency.

Perfusion: The delivery of fluid to through the bloodstream to an organ or tissue.

Peri-: Surrounding.

Pero-: Deformed.

-pexy: Surgical fixation.

Pharynx: Throat.

-pheresis: Removal.

Phlebo-: Vein.

-phore: Processor.

Phot(o): Light.

-physis: Growth.

-piesis: Pressure.

Pituitary gland: The main endocrine gland that hormones that control other glands.

-plasm: Formation.

Plasma: The liquid part of blood.

-plasty: Surgical repair.

Platelets: The part of blood that causes clotting to help stop bleeding.

Pleura: A membrane around the lungs.

-pnea: Breathing.

Pneum(o): Lungs, respiration.

Poly-: Much, many.

Por(o): Passage.

Prim-: First.

Pro-: Before.

Prognosis: A forecast for what is believed to be the most likely scenario for the outcome of a disease.

Prone: Lying on the abdomen.

Pulmonary: Relating to the lungs.

Q

Quadriceps muscle: Muscle group in the thigh.

Quadriplegia: Partial or total paralysis of the limbs and torso.

Quasi: Resemblance.

R

Radicul(o): Nerve root.

REM sleep: A stage of sleep that is characterized by rapid eye movement.

Resuscitation: The revival of someone or something from alleged death or unconsciousness.

Retina: Sensory membrane that coats the back of the eye. It sends images of what the eyes see to the brain.

Rickets: A condition in children characterized by a softening and weakening of the bones.

Rigor mortis: Postmortem rigidity of the muscles and joints that typically sets in several hours after death.

Rotator cuff: A group of tendons that provide stability for the shoulder joint.

-rrhage: Excessive discharge.

-rrhaphy: Suture.

-rrhexis: Rupture.

S

Sciatic nerve: The largest nerve in the body that begins at the nerve roots in the lumbar section of the spinal cord.

Sciatica: Pain that is felt along the sciatic nerve and can run down the back of the thigh.

Scler-: Hard.

Sclera: The white part of the eye.

Scoli(o): Crooked.

-scopy: Viewing process.

Scot(o): Darkness.

Scurvy: Disorder of the blood vessels characterized by bleeding gums, bleeding under the skin, and extreme weakness.

Seizure: A sudden, uncontrolled surge of electrical activity in the brain that can cause convulsion.

Serum: Clear liquid that can be parted from clotted blood.

Somatic: Relating to the body.

Spectr-: Image.

Sphen(o): Wedge-shaped.

Spin(o): Spine.

Spir(o): To breathe.

Spleen: A very vascular organ that is found in the abdominal region that makes lymphocytes.

Spondyl(o): Vertebra.

Squamous Cell Carcinoma: A skin cancer that typically occurs as a result of regularly exposed sunlight or other types of ultraviolet radiation.

-stalsis: Contraction.

-stasis: Maintaining a certain level.

-stenosis: Abnormal narrowing.

Stere(o): Three dimensional.

Stom(o): Mouth.

-stomy: New opening.

Start(i): Layer.

Strept(o): Twisted.

-stroma: Supportive tissue of an organ.

Sucrose: Cane or beet sugar.

Supine: Lying on back.

Synaps(o): Point of contact.

Systolic blood pressure: The first number in a blood pressure reading.

T

Tachy-: Fast.

Tal(o): Ankle.

Taut-: Same.

Tax(o): Coordination.

Tel(o): Complete.

Tela: A tissue or layer of tissue.

Tele(o): End.

Temp(o): Time.

Tendon: A cord of dense connective tissue that joins a muscle with another body part.

Therm(o): Heat.

Thoracic: Pertaining to the thorax.

Thorax: Body part that is located between the neck and the abdominal region.

Thromb(o): Blood clot.

Thyroid: A gland that produces and stores hormones that help control blood pressure, heart rate, body temperature, and the rate at which food is transformed into energy.

Tibia: One of the bones of the lower leg.

-tic: Relating to.

Tinnitus: The sensation of a ringing sound or some other noise in the ears.

Tissue: A group of cells.

Tom(o): Slice.

-tomy: Incision.

Topical: Relating to a specific area.

Tors(o): Twisted.

Tox(o): Poison.

Trachea: Wind pipe, which runs down the larynx.

Trans-: Through.

Transfusion: The process of transferring blood from one person to another.

Tremor: Involuntary shaking of body parts.

Triceps: A three-headed muscle at the back of the upper arm.

Trich(o): Hair.

-trophic: Nutrition.

-trophy: Development.

-tropic: Turning.

Tumescence: Swelling:

U

Ulcer: A lesion that erodes an organ or tissue.

-ule: Little.

Ultra-: Beyond.

-um: Structure.

Umbilicus: Navel.

Ungual: Relating to the nails.

V

Varicose veins: Twisted veins that are often visible through the skin.

Vas(o): Vessel.

Ventr(o): Front.

Ventricles: The heart chambers that accept blood from the atria and send it to the systemic and pulmonary circulatory systems.

Vertebrae: Bones or segments that compose the spinal column.

Viscer(o): Body organs.

Viscera: Organs in the body's cavity.

Vit(o): Life.

Vivi-: Alive.

W

Whey: The watery part of milk that gets separated from the curds after the process of coagulation.

Whooping cough: A respiratory disease characterized by a convulsive cough. It is acute and very contagious.

X

Xen(o): Foreign.

Xer(o): Dry.

Xerophthalmia: Very dry eyes due to malfunctioning tear glands.

Y

YO: Years old.

Z

Zyg(o): Yoke.

Zygoma: Cheekbone.

Body Systems

Cardiovascular System

Arteries, veins, capillaries, blood, and heart.

Digestive System

Esophagus, gallbladder, large intestine, liver, pancreas, salivary glands, small intestine, stomach, teeth, and tongue.

Endocrine System

Adrenal glands, gonads, hormones, pancreas, pituitary gland, and thyroid.

Integumentary System

Glands in skin, hair, nails, and skin.

Lymphatic System

Lymph fluid, lymph nodes, lymphatic vessels, spleen, thymus, and tonsils.

Muscular System

Muscles and tendons.

Nervous System

Brain, ganglia, nerves, sensory organs, and spinal cord.

Reproductive System

Genitalia

Males: Ducts, prostate, testes, and urethra.

Females: Ovaries, uterine tubes, and uterus.

Respiratory System

Bronchi, larynx, lungs, pharynx, nose, and trachea.

Sensory System

Ears, eyes, mouth, nose, and skin receptors.

Skeletal System

Bones and joints.

Urinary

Bladder, kidneys, ureters, and urethra.

<u>Closing</u>

The understanding and memorization of medical terminology comes with experience. The more you practice, the more experienced you will become.

But consistency is also important.

It makes little sense to study hard for twelve hours a day for two days straight and then take the next five days off after that.

People are typically better off studying a little bit at a time on a regular basis, rather than trying to do it all at once on an infrequent basis.

Start with the terms that are likely to be more commonly used than others in the medical field.

To help determine which terms are more widely used than others, think back to your own experiences.

If you have been to various doctors over the years and have heard them using the term, "ITIS" on more than one occasion, chances are that it's one of the more popular terms.

www.ingramcontent.com/pod-product-compliance
Lightning Source LLC
Chambersburg PA
CBHW030737180526
45157CB00008BA/3211